Good Food Motivation

By Rita Ferdinando

Start Keeping Track!

Get Motivated

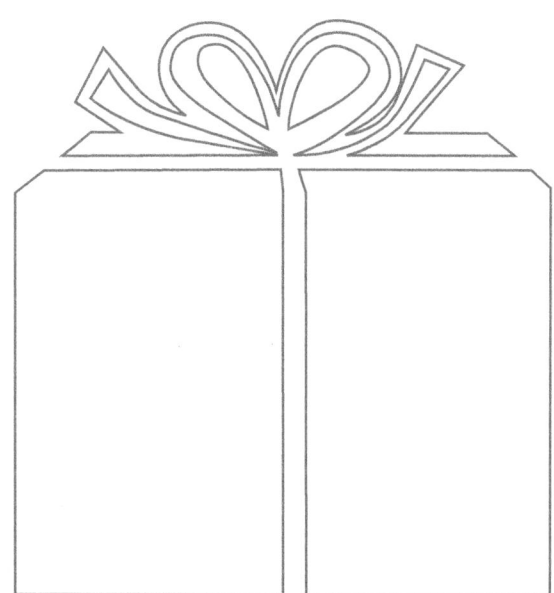

A c k n o w l e d g e m e n t s : *This Book Was Written So That You Will Have The Motivation To Eat Healthy!*

Food Motivation
"Feeling Better Already"

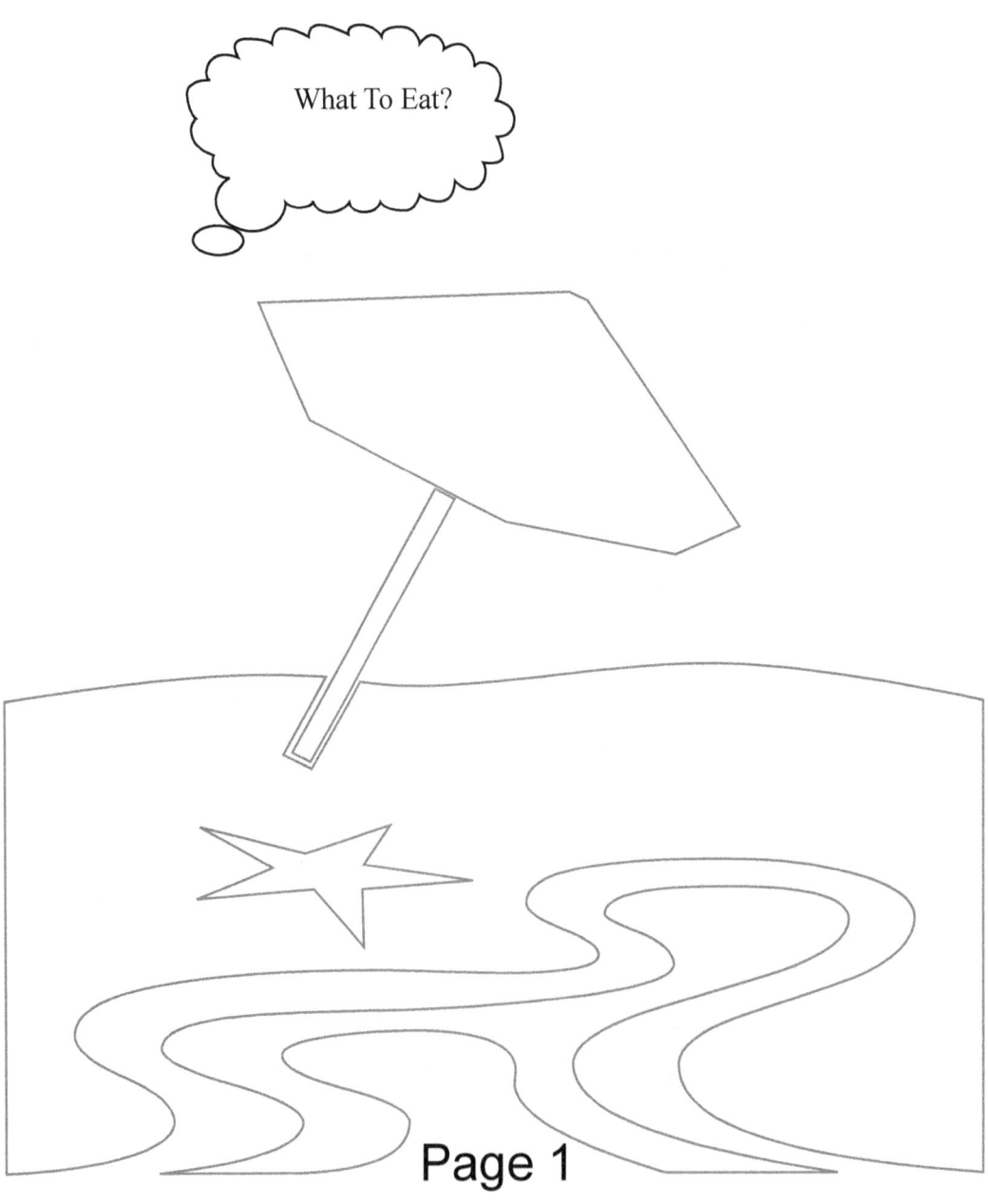

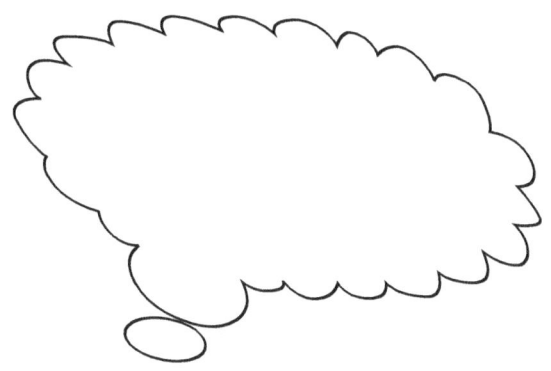

You know the old saying apple keeps the Doctor away!

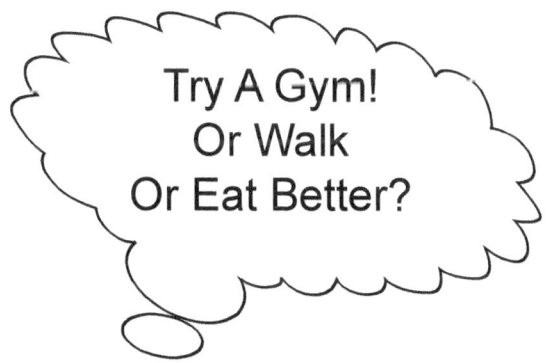

Try A Gym!
Or Walk
Or Eat Better?

Good Food
Or Bad Food

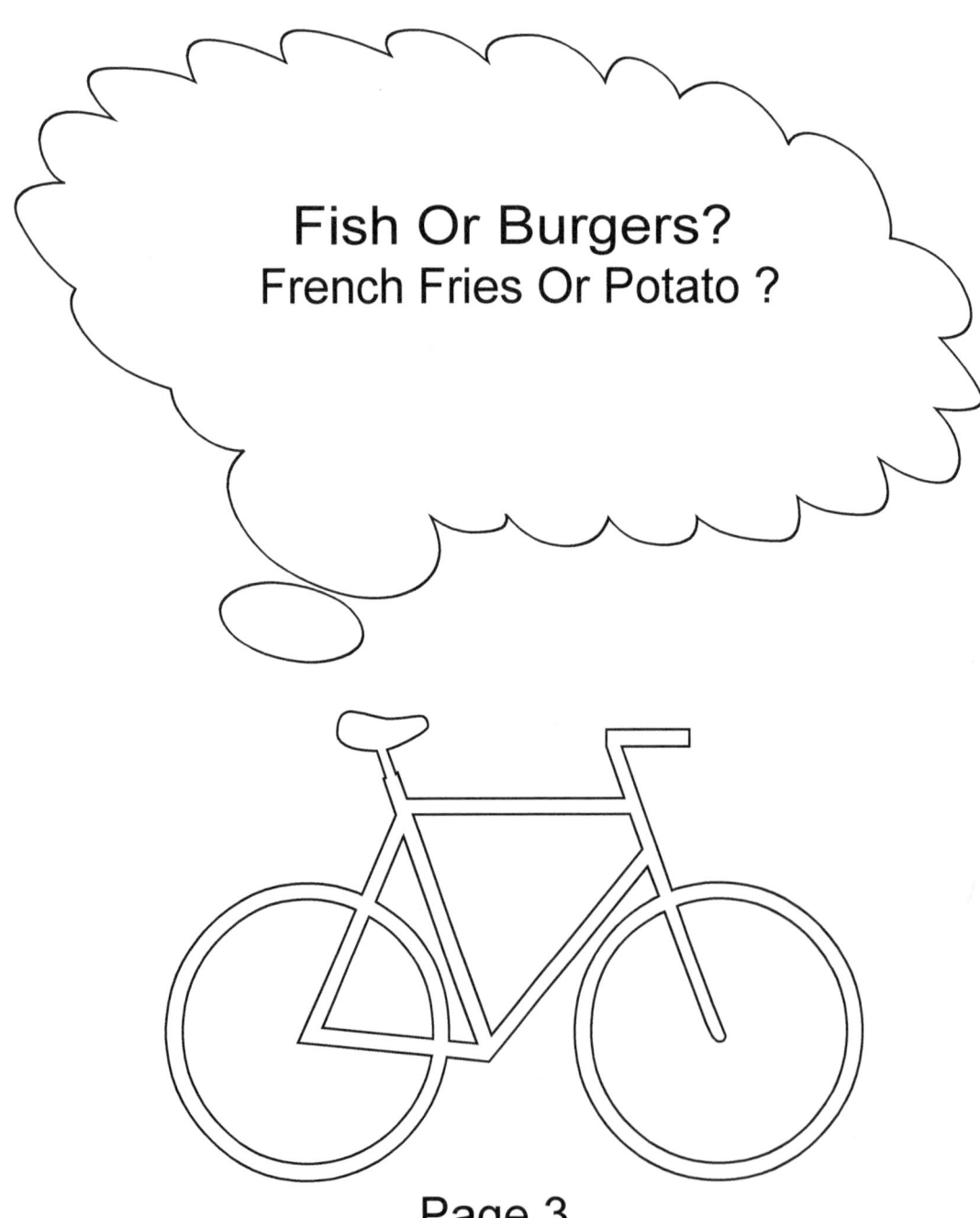

Fish Or Burgers?
French Fries Or Potato ?

Good Choices

Fish
Sweet Potato
Hotdogs
Eggs
Salad
Fruit

Nuts Or Soup!

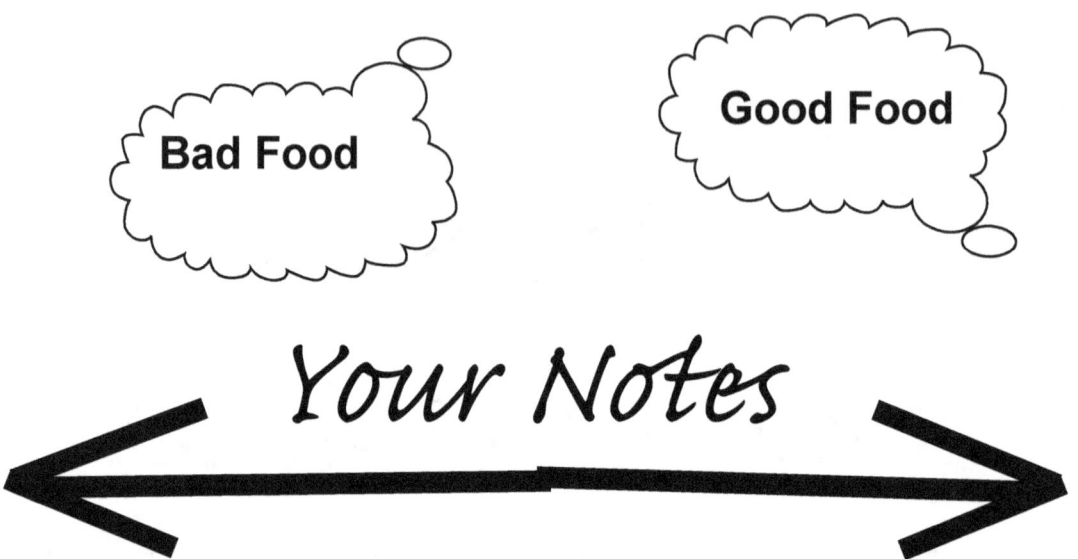

Water or Soda ?

Are You Counting Calories?
Which is more Healthy ?

Consult with your Dietition
Ask your Doctor for a List.

Start Planning
Breakfast
Lunch
Dinner
Snacks

When Do I see the doctor again!

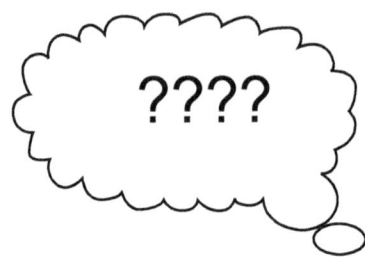

Your Notes

Eating Better

Monday
Tuesday
Wednesday
Thursday
Friday
Saturday
Sunday

What Are You Eating?

Your Notes

Breakfast ?

Your Notes

Your Notes

Lunch ?

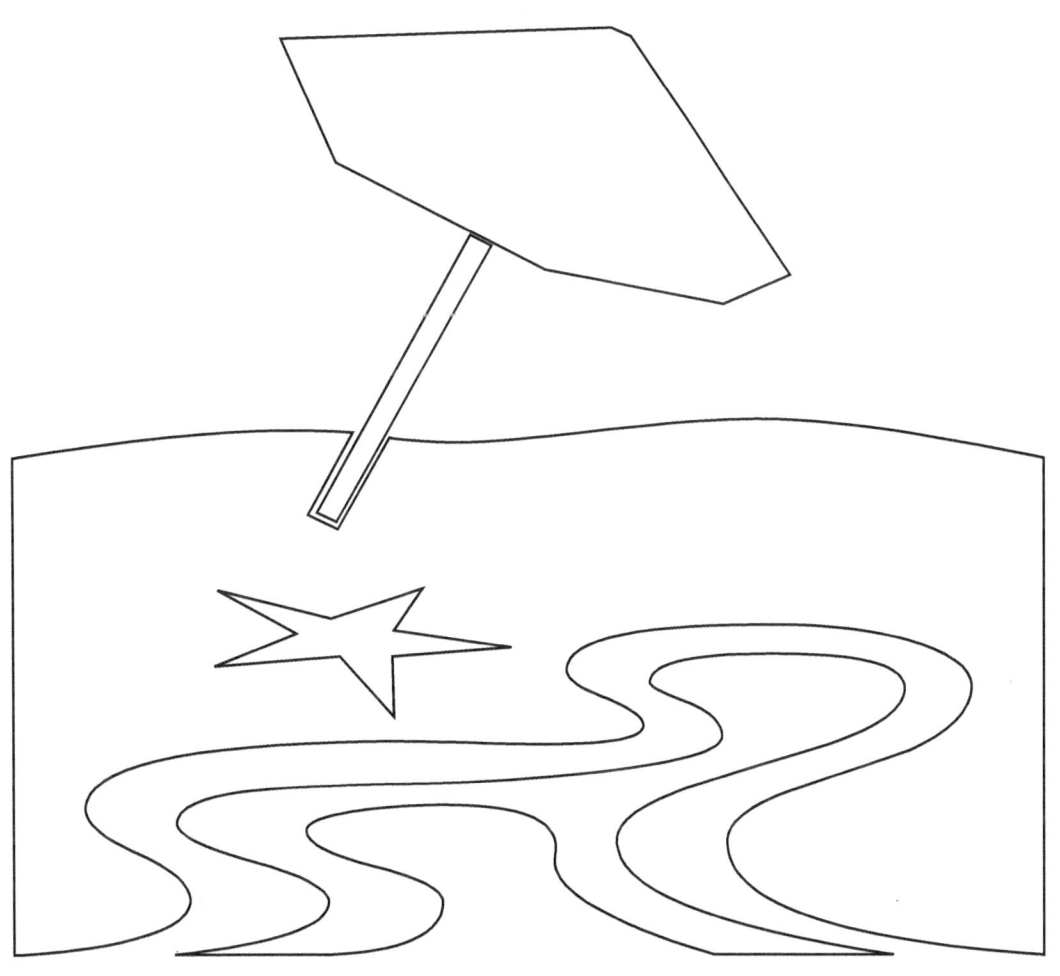

Lunch ?

Your Notes

Dinner ?

Your Notes

Dinner ?

Dinner ?

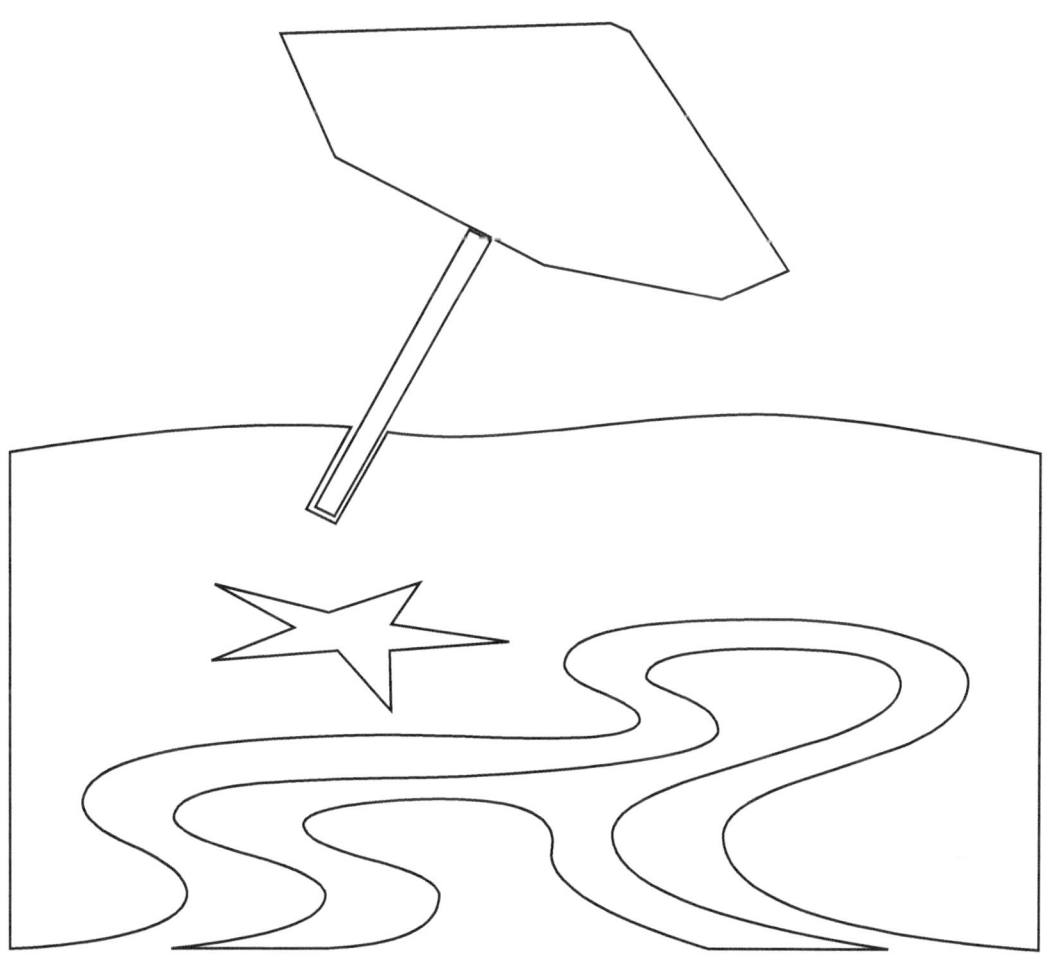

Your Notes

Snacks ?

Your Notes

Lite Exercise

Your Notes

Snacks

Your Notes

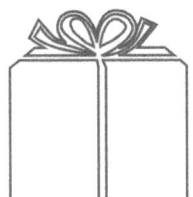

www.ingramcontent.com/pod-product-compliance
Lightning Source LLC
Chambersburg PA
CBHW080532190526
45169CB00008B/3126